Table of Contents

Introduction 3
   Testosterone 3
   Low Testosterone Levels 4
   Testing Testosterone 5
   Testosterone Replacement Therapy 6
   Testosterone Imbalances 7
Testosterone Levels And Aging 10
   Treatment 12
   Testosterone-Boosting Foods 15
   Foods That May Reduce Testosterone 21
Recipes 25
   Spice-Rubbed Chicken With Pomegranate Salad 25
   Spelt & Wild Mushroom Risotto 27
   Spicy Spaghetti With Garlic Mushrooms 28
   Carrot, Lentil & Orange Soup 29
   Leek, Potato & Bacon Bake 31
   Lamb Meatball & Pea Pilaf 32
   Pan-Fried Venison With Blackberry Sauce 33
   Spiced Chicken With Rice & Crisp Red Onions 35
   Prawn Sweet Chilli Noodle Salad 36
   Chargrilled Turkey With Quinoa Tabbouleh & Tahini Dressing 37

Chicken Korma 39

Oven-Baked Fish & Chips 42

Chicken, Edamame & Ginger Pilaf 43

Spiced Turkey With Bulgur & Pomegranate Salad 44

Summer Pea Pasta 47

Miso Steak 48

Low-Fat Roasties 49

Mushroom & Thyme Risotto 51

Mango & Passion Fruit Meringue Roulade 52

Chicken With Lemon & Courgette Couscous 54

Thai Red Duck With Sticky Pineapple Rice 55

Prawn, Fennel & Rocket Risotto 57

Red Lentil, Chickpea & Chilli Soup 58

Granola 60

Cauliflower Mac and Cheese 62

Balsamic And Bacon Vegetable Medley 63

Garden Vegetable Soup 65

French Onion Soup 67

Blueberry Muffin Cake 68

Pecan Cookie 70

Introduction

Some foods, including soy, dairy, and specific fats, may lower testosterone levels in the body. However, a person can also increase testosterone levels naturally, by exercising regularly and maintaining a healthful weight. The food a person eats can affect many aspects of their health, not just their waistline. Food powers the cells and may affect some of the body's other components, including hormones, such as testosterone. Consuming too much of certain foods may throw the body's hormones out of balance or make it more difficult for the body to use hormones correctly. This contains information about testosterone, diet and recipes.

Testosterone

Testosterone is a hormone found in humans, as well as in other animals. The testicles primarily make testosterone in men. Women's ovaries also make testosterone, though in much smaller amounts. The production of testosterone starts to increase significantly during puberty, and begins to dip after age 30 or so. Testosterone is most often associated with sex drive, and plays a vital role in sperm production. It also affects bone and muscle mass, the way men store fat in the body, and even red blood cell production. A man's testosterone levels can also affect his mood.

Low Testosterone Levels

Low levels of testosterone, also called low T levels, can produce a variety of symptoms in men, including:

- decreased sex drive

- less energy

- weight gain

- feelings of depression

- moodiness

- low self-esteem

- less body hair

- thinner bones

While testosterone production naturally tapers off as a man ages, other factors can cause hormone levels to drop. Injury to the testicles and cancer treatments such as chemotherapy or radiation can negatively affect testosterone production. Chronic health conditions and stress can also reduce testosterone production. Some of these include:

- AIDS

- kidney disease

- alcoholism

- cirrhosis of the liver

Testing Testosterone

A simple blood test can determine testosterone levels. There's a wide range of normal or healthy levels of testosterone circulating in the bloodstream. The normal range of testosterone for men is between 280 and 1,100 nanograms per deciliter (ng/dL) for adult males, and between 15 and 70 ng/dL for adult females, according to the University of Rochester Medical Center. Ranges can vary among different labs, so it's important to speak with your doctor about your results. If an adult male's testosterone levels are below 300 ng/dL, a doctor may do a workup to determine the cause of low testosterone, according to the American Urological Association. Low testosterone levels could be a sign of pituitary gland problems. The pituitary gland sends a signaling hormone to the testicles to produce more testosterone. A low T test result in an adult man could mean the pituitary gland isn't working properly. But a young teen with low testosterone levels might be experiencing delayed puberty. Moderately elevated testosterone levels in men tend to produce few noticeable symptoms. Boys with higher levels of testosterone may begin puberty earlier. Women with higher than normal testosterone may develop masculine features. Abnormally high levels of testosterone could be the result of an adrenal gland disorder, or even cancer of the testes. High testosterone levels may also occur in less serious conditions. For example, congenital adrenal hyperplasia, which can affect males and females, is a rare but natural cause for elevated testosterone production. If your testosterone levels are extremely high, your doctor may order other tests to find out the cause.

Testosterone Replacement Therapy

Reduced testosterone production, a condition known as hypogonadism, doesn't always require treatment. You may be a candidate for testosterone replacement therapy if low T is interfering with your health and quality of life. Artificial testosterone can be administered orally, through injections, or with gels or patches on the skin. Replacement therapy may produce desired results, such as greater muscle mass and a stronger sex drive. But the treatment does carry some side effects. These include:

- oily skin
- fluid retention
- testicles shrinking
- decrease in sperm production

Some studies have found no greater risk of prostate cancer with testosterone replacement therapy, but it continues to be a topic of ongoing research. One study suggests that there's a lower risk of aggressive prostate cancers for those on testosterone replacement therapy, but more research is needed. Research shows little evidence of abnormal or unhealthy psychological changes in men receiving supervised testosterone therapy to treat their low T, according to a 2009 study in the journal Therapeutics and Clinical Risk Management.

Testosterone Imbalances
High or low levels of testosterone can lead to dysfunction in the parts of the body normally regulated by the hormone.

When a man has low testosterone, or hypogonadism, he may experience:

- reduced sex drive

- erectile dysfunction

- low sperm count

- enlarged or swollen breast tissue

Over time, these symptoms may develop in the following ways:

- loss of body hair

- loss of muscle bulk

- loss of strength

- increased body fat

Chronic, or ongoing, low testosterone may lead to osteoporosis, mood swings, reduced energy, and testicular shrinkage. Causes can include:

- testicular injury, such as castration

- infection of the testicles

- medications, such as opiate analgesics
- disorders that affect the hormones, such as pituitary tumors or high prolactin levels
- chronic diseases, including type 2 diabetes, kidney and liver disease, obesity, and HIV/AIDS
- genetic diseases, such as Klinefelter syndrome, Prader-Willi syndrome, hemochromatosis, Kallman syndrome, and myotonic dystrophy

Too much testosterone, on the other hand, can lead to the triggering of puberty before the age of 9 years. This condition would mainly affect younger men and is much rarer. In women, however, high testosterone levels can lead to male pattern baldness, a deep voice, and menstrual irregularities, as well as:

- growth and swelling of the clitoris
- changes in body shape
- reduction in breast size
- oily skin
- acne

- facial hair growth around the body, lips, and chin

Recent studies have also linked high testosterone levels in women to the risk of uterine fibroids. Testosterone imbalances can be detected with a blood test and treated accordingly.

Testosterone Levels And Aging

Testosterone levels naturally decrease as a man ages. The effects of gradually lowering testosterone levels as men age have received increasing attention in recent years. It is known as late-onset hypogonadism. After the age of 40, the concentration of circulating testosterone falls by about 1.6 percent every year for most men. By the age of 60, the low levels of testosterone would lead to a diagnosis of hypogonadism in younger men. About 4 in 10 men have hypogonadism by the time they reach 45 years old. The number of cases in which older men have been diagnosed as having low testosterone increased 170 percent since 2012. Low testosterone has been associated with increased mortality in male veterans. Late-onset hypogonadism has become a recognized medical condition, although many of the symptoms are associated with normal aging. The following are symptoms of late-onset hypogonadism:

- diminished erectile quality, particularly at night
- decreased libido
- mood changes
- reduced cognitive function
- fatigue, depression, and anger
- a decrease in muscle mass and strength
- decreased body hair
- skin changes
- decreased bone mass and bone mineral density
- increase in abdominal fat mass

As well as sexual dysfunction, late-onset hypogonadism has also been associated with metabolic disease and cardiovascular disease. The degree to which testosterone levels decline varies between men, but a growing number of men experience the effects of reduced testosterone levels. Life expectancy has increased, and many men now live beyond the age of 60 years. As a result, a higher number of men see the effects of age-related testosterone depletion.

Treatment

Administering treatment for hypogonadism as the result of a disease differs from treating late-onset hypogonadism in older men.

Testosterone supplements

One proposed treatment for low testosterone comes in the form of testosterone supplements. One type of testosterone supplement, methyltestosterone, has received approval from the United States Food and Drug Administration (FDA). However, guidelines advise doctors not to prescribe this supplement due to the speed with which the liver metabolizes testosterone. This can lead to liver toxicity. While doctors can legally prescribe the supplement, they generally try to avoid this. Until stronger evidence is available to support the benefits and safety of testosterone supplementation, only older adults with severe clinical symptoms of low testosterone should be candidates for these supplements. The FDA have advised that testosterone supplements are not suitable to treat late-onset hypogonadism, and a doctor should only prescribe them for an identifiable cause.

Testosterone replacement therapy

Testosterone replacement therapy (TRT) can help restore some affected functions of low testosterone. Studies have shown that TRT mainly impacts bone strength and hemoglobin levels in the blood, but not mental sharpness. The treatment can be administered by:

- skin gels and patches

- injections

- tablets that are absorbed through the gums

These can, however, trigger side effects, including:

- increased red blood cell count

- prostate and breast enlargement

- acne

- in rare cases, breathing difficulties during sleep

- increased risk of cardiovascular disease, although this is subject to debate

Deciding to pursue a course of TRT involves deciding between the perceived benefit of the therapy on the symptoms of a particular individual and the risks of the treatment. A recent study, for example, suggests that TRT provides extra benefit for overall mortality and stroke for men whose testosterone levels have normalized with TRT. However, the Endocrine Society advises that doctors should not prescribe TRT to men aged less than 65 years, even if they have low testosterone levels. The risks and suggested benefits of TRT for men younger than this are unclear, as are the benefits. Current research is conflicting. Additional studies into testosterone replacement are necessary for physicians to fully understand its potential risks and benefits, and to identify the individuals that may see the most benefit.

Prohormone supplements and heart disease

Prohormones are a variety of steroid. They are often used to support weight loss and muscle-building. A number of prohormone supplements are marketed at men to treat low testosterone levels. Such supplements can include dehydroepiandrosterone (DHEA), and the herbal product Tribulus terrestris. However, a bill was passed in 2014 banning designer anabolic steroids. Legal variants have emerged since. However, there is little, if any, research to indicate that these prohormone supplements affect testosterone levels. Research from 2016 did not find any evidence that Tribulus terrestris, for example, can increase testosterone levels. Such remedies may pose a risk to health. The law does not require herbal supplements to be proven safe before sale, so caution is advised. Prohormones can increase testosterone but boost estrogen, the female hormone, at the same time. They can also cause an imbalance in blood cholesterol, decreasing levels of "good" cholesterol. The potential side effects of prohormones plus their unproven clinical benefits make them a poor, possibly dangerous choice for boosting testosterone.

Testosterone-Boosting Foods
A person with low testosterone may benefit from trying:

Ginger

People have used ginger for medicinal and culinary purposes for centuries. Modern research indicates that this root may improve fertility in men. According to the findings of a 2012 study, taking a daily ginger supplement for 3 months increased testosterone levels by 17.7 percent in a group of 75 adult male participants with fertility issues. The authors suggested that ginger may also improve sperm health in other ways. Authors of a study from 2013 report that ginger increased testosterone and antioxidant levels in a diabetic rat model in just 30 days.

Oysters

Oysters contain more zinc per serving than any other food — and zinc is important for sperm health and reproductive function. Males with severe zinc deficiency may develop hypogonadism, in which the body does not produce enough testosterone. They may also experience impotence or delayed sexual maturation. People can also find the mineral in:

• other shellfish

• red meat

• poultry

- beans

- nuts

It is important to note that zinc and copper compete for absorption. Take care when choosing supplements to avoid consuming too much of either mineral.

Pomegranates

The pomegranate is an age-old symbol of fertility and sexual function, and its antioxidant levels may support heart health and stress reduction. Also, results of a study from 2012 indicate that pomegranate may boost testosterone levels in men and women. Sixty healthy participants drank pure pomegranate juice for 14 days, and researchers tested the levels of testosterone in their saliva three times a day. At the end of the study period, both male and female participants displayed an average 24 percent increase in salivary testosterone levels. They also experienced improvements in mood and blood pressure.

Fortified plant milks

Vitamin D is an essential nutrient, and results of a study from 2011 suggest that it may increase testosterone levels in men. It is important to note that the dosage in this study was 3,332 international units (IU) of the vitamin per day, which far exceeds the 400 IU recommended daily for healthy people. While sun exposure is one of the best ways to get vitamin D, not everyone can spend enough time outdoors in sunny weather. In the average American diet, fortified foods provide the majority of the vitamin D. Many plant milks, such as those made from almonds, soy, hemp, and flax, contain 25 percent of a person's vitamin D requirement per serving. However, it is always best to verify nutritional contents by checking labeling. Research has put to rest the concern that soy lowers testosterone levels — the bulk of the evidence shows that soy does not have this effect. Also, some manufacturers fortify the following with vitamin D:

• milk and other dairy products

• orange juice

• cereals

The medical community is not convinced that vitamin D boosts testosterone levels in healthy people. A study from 2017, for example, found that the vitamin had no such effect. It is important to remember, however, that getting enough vitamin D every day is essential for overall health.

Leafy green vegetables

Vegetables such as spinach, Swiss chard, and kale are rich in magnesium, a mineral that may increase the body's level of testosterone. Authors of a study from 2011 found that taking magnesium supplements for 4 weeks prompted an increase in testosterone levels of sedentary participants and those who were athletes. The testosterone increases were greater, however, in the active participants. Other good dietary sources of magnesium are:

• beans and lentils

• nuts and seeds

• whole grains

Fatty fish and fish oil

The United States Department of Agriculture recommend that people eat seafood twice weekly. Fatty fish may be especially beneficial because they are rich in omega-3 fatty acids. A person can also boost their fatty acid levels by taking fish oil or omega-3 supplements. Results of an animal-based study from 2016 indicate that fish oil can increase the quality of semen and the serum testosterone levels in dogs by improving their fatty acid profiles. A study in mice reported similar findings. Examples of fish that are rich in omega-3 fatty acids include:

- Atlantic mackerel

- herring

- salmon

- sardines

- trout

Extra-virgin olive oil

Olive oil is a staple of the Mediterranean diet, which may have many health benefits, including a reduced risk of heart disease and cancer. The oil is rich in monounsaturated fat and vitamin E, an antioxidant. These factors likely contribute to the food's health benefits. Extra-virgin olive oil may also improve male reproductive health. Results of a small-scale study indicate that the oil may boost serum testosterone levels in healthy adult men. Participants also experienced an increase in luteinizing hormone, which stimulates cells in the testes to produce testosterone.

Onions

Onions may provide many health benefits, from supporting the heart to slimming the waistline. They are also good sources of several nutrients and antioxidants. In addition, onions may increase low levels of testosterone. In a 2012 study with a rat model, researchers found that a daily intake of fresh onion juice for 4 weeks significantly increased serum total testosterone levels. However, determining the effects in humans will require further research.

Foods That May Reduce Testosterone
Soy products

Soy foods, such as tofu, edamame, and soy protein isolates, contain phytoestrogens. These compounds are physically similar to the estrogen in the body and function in a similar way. A study in the journal German Medical Science notes that although scientists have carried out a lot of research into soy, they still do not understand it fully. The paper notes that many studies have not found a connection between eating soy products and altered serum testosterone or estrogen levels. However, another study showed that breast tenderness and estrogen concentrations returned to normal after a man stopped using soy. The researchers suggested that phytoestrogens in soy might affect the body without changing the body's hormone levels, which could cause symptoms of high estrogen. Researchers need to do more high-quality research in both males and females to identify the exact effects of soy in the body.

Dairy products

Many people looking to raise their testosterone levels might choose to avoid dairy products. This may be because some cow's milk contains synthetic or natural hormones, which might affect a person's testosterone levels. Also, animal feed may contain soy, which could increase the levels of estrogen in the cow's milk.

Alcohol

Anyone with concerns about their testosterone levels might also consider giving up or limiting drinking alcohol. This may be especially true for males. While some studies have found evidence that a small amount of alcohol increases testosterone levels in men, this is generally not the case. As a study posted to Current Drug Abuse Review notes, heavy drinking or regular drinking over long periods causes a decrease of testosterone in males. The paper also notes that alcohol consumption causes an increase in testosterone levels in women.

Mint

Peppermint and spearmint may make a calming tea, but the menthol in mint may reduce testosterone levels. According to a study paper in Advanced Pharmaceutical Bulletin, scientists treated female rats with polycystic ovarian syndrome (PCOS) with spearmint essential oil to test its effects on the disorder. Researchers noted that spearmint essential oil reduced testosterone levels in these rats. A review posted to BMC Complementary & Alternative Medicine also noted that there is some high-quality evidence showing that mint lowers testosterone levels in women with PCOS. However, there is not enough high-quality evidence surrounding the effect of the herb in general. Most of the research on the topic focuses on animal models or women. Future studies should investigate the effects of mint in both sexes to get a better overall picture.

Bread, pastries, and desserts

A study in the journal Nutrients linked a diet high in bread, pastries, and other desserts to low total testosterone levels in Taiwanese men. Additional factors included high dairy consumption, eating out regularly, and not eating enough dark green vegetables. According to the article, these men also had decreased muscle mass and increased body fat.

Licorice root

A study in Integrative Medicine Research notes that licorice root can reduce testosterone in healthy women during menstrual cycles. Animal studies also show that licorice supplementation can reduce testosterone levels. Ideally, any future studies would look into the effects of licorice on both sexes to better understand how the herb acts in general.

Certain fats

The type of fat a person eats may also affect their testosterone levels and function. A study in the Asian Journal of Andrology looked at the dietary patterns of young, healthy men in regards to their hormone levels and testicular function. Their research indicated that eating trans fats may lower testosterone levels in the body. They also found that too many omega-6 fatty acids appear to reduce testicular size and function. However, eating plenty of polyunsaturated omega-3 fatty acids may increase testicle size and improve function. The researchers called for more studies to confirm their findings, but people who are worried about their testosterone levels may want to avoid trans fats and limit omega-6 fats.

Recipes
Spice-Rubbed Chicken With Pomegranate Salad
Ingredients

- 4 skinless chicken leg joints, cut into drumsticks and thighs

- 2½ tsp turmeric

- 2½ tsp sweet paprika

- ½ tsp chilli flakes

- 2½ tsp coarsely ground black pepper

- 1 tbsp olive oil

- 3 tbsp white wine vinegar

For the salad

- seeds from 1 pomegranate
- 3 oranges, segmented
- juice ½ lime, plus extra wedges to serve
- 1 tbsp pomegranate molasses
- small handful mint leaves, torn

Method

- Score the chicken with a sharp knife, about 2-3 cuts in each piece. Mix the spices with a little salt, the olive oil and vinegar in a small bowl. Using gloves (turmeric stains your fingers), rub this spice mixture over the chicken pieces and transfer to a roasting tin. Leave to marinate for at least 20 mins, or overnight in the fridge if you're preparing ahead.

- Heat oven to 200C/180C fan/gas 6. Cover the chicken with foil and bake for 30 mins. Remove the foil and continue cooking in the oven for another 10 mins until tender. Baste with tin juices and rest for 5 mins before serving.

- Meanwhile, make the salad. Mix the pomegranate seeds with the orange segments, mix the lime juice with the pomegranate molasses, then drizzle over. Scatter with torn mint leaves and serve alongside the chicken.

Spelt & Wild Mushroom Risotto
Ingredients

- 200g pearled spelt

- 25g dried porcini mushrooms

- ½ tbsp olive oil

- 1 onion, finely diced

- 2 garlic cloves, finely chopped

- 100g chestnut button mushroom, cut into quarters

- 100ml white wine

- 1l hot vegetable stock

- 1 tbsp low-fat crème fraîche

- bunch chives, finely chopped

- handful grated pecorino or parmesan to serve (optional)

Method

- Cover the spelt with cold water and soak the dried mushrooms in 100ml boiling water in a separate bowl for 20 mins. Heat the olive oil in a large frying pan. Tip in the onion and garlic, cook for 2 mins, then add the chestnut mushrooms and cook for a further 2 mins. Drain the spelt and add along with the wine. Simmer until almost all the liquid evaporates, stirring often.

- Drain the porcini mushrooms, add them to the pan and the soaking liquid to the vegetable stock. Stir in the stock 1 cup at a time and simmer, stirring often, until all liquid is absorbed and the spelt is just tender, about 20 mins in total. Stir in the crème fraîche and season with salt and pepper. Spoon onto plates and sprinkle over chives and cheese (if using).

Spicy Spaghetti With Garlic Mushrooms
Ingredients

- 2 tbsp olive oil

- 250g pack chestnut mushroom, thickly sliced

- 1 garlic clove, thinly sliced

- small bunch parsley, leaves only

- 1 celery stick, finely chopped

- 1 onion, finely chopped

- 400g can chopped tomato

- 1/2 red chilli, deseeded and finely chopped, (or use drieds chilli flakes)

- 300g spaghetti

Method

- Heat 1 tbsp oil in a pan, add the mushrooms, then fry over a high heat for 3 mins until golden and softened. Add the garlic, fry for 1 min more, then tip into a bowl with the parsley. Add the onion and celery to the pan with the rest of the oil, then fry for 5 mins until lightly coloured.

- Stir in the tomatoes, chilli and a little salt, then bring to the boil. Reduce the heat and simmer, uncovered, for 10 mins until thickened. Meanwhile, boil the spaghetti, then drain. Toss with the sauce, top with the garlicky mushrooms, then serve.

Carrot, Lentil & Orange Soup
Ingredients

- 1 tsp cumin seeds

- 2 tsp coriander seeds

- 1 onion chopped

- 225g carrots diced

- 75g red lentils

- 300ml orange juice

- 2 tbsp low-fat natural yogurt

- fresh chopped coriander to garnish

- pinch paprika to garnish

- 600ml vegetable stock

Method

- Crush the seeds in a pestle and mortar, then dry-fry for 2 mins in a large pan until lightly browned. Add the onion, carrots, lentils, orange juice, stock and seasoning, then bring to the boil. Cover and simmer for 30 mins until the lentils are soft.

- Transfer to a food processor in batches and process until smooth. Return to the pan, then gently reheat, stirring occasionally. Adjust seasoning to taste. Ladle into individual serving bowls, swirl the yogurt over and sprinkle with the chopped coriander leaves and paprika. Serve immediately.

Leek, Potato & Bacon Bake
Ingredients

- 600ml chicken or vegetable stock

- 1kg potato, thinly sliced

- 6 leeks, thinly sliced into rounds

- 25g butter

- 3-4 rashers streaky bacon, snipped

- 3 tbsp double cream (optional)

Method

- Heat oven to 200C/fan 180C/gas 6. Put the stock in a large pan, bring to the boil, then add the potatoes and the leeks. Bring back to the boil for 5 mins, then drain well, reserving the stock in a jug.

- Meanwhile, butter a large baking dish. Layer up the potatoes and leeks, seasoning as you go, then scatter the bacon over the top. Season well, pour over 200ml of the reserved stock, then spoon over the cream (if using) and cover with foil. Can be made up to 1 day ahead and chilled. Bake for 40 mins, uncovering halfway through so that the bacon crisps.

Lamb Meatball & Pea Pilaf

Ingredients

- 400g pack lean minced lamb

- 3 garlic cloves, crushed

- 2 tsp cumin

- 300g basmati rice

- enough lamb or vegetable stock to cover the rice, from a cube is fine

- 300g frozen pea

- zest 2 lemon, juice of 1

For the cucumber yogurt

- 1/2 cucumber, finely chopped or grated

- 150ml pot mild natural yogurt

- small bunch mint, leaves torn

Method

- Mix the lamb with half the garlic and 1 tsp of the cumin, then season and shape into about 16 balls – it's easier if you wet your hands. Heat a large frying pan (with a lid for later), then fry the meatballs for about 8 mins until golden and cooked through. Remove from the pan, set aside, then tip in the rice, final tsp of cumin and remaining garlic. Fry for 30 secs, stirring, then pour in enough stock to cover. Cover and simmer for 10 mins or until almost all of the liquid is absorbed.

- Stir in the peas, return the meatballs to the pan, then warm through for a few mins until the peas are tender. Meanwhile mix the cucumber, yogurt and half the mint together, then season. To finish the pilaf, stir in the lemon zest and juice with some seasoning and the remaining mint. Serve with a good dollop of the cooling cucumber yogurt.

Pan-Fried Venison With Blackberry Sauce
Ingredients

- 1 tbsp olive oil

- 2 thick venison steaks, or 4 medallions

- 1 tbsp balsamic vinegar

- 150ml beef stock (made with 2 tsp Knorr Touch of Taste beef concentrate)

- 2 tbsp redcurrant jelly

- 1 garlic clove, crushed

- 85g fresh or frozen blackberry

Method

- Heat the oil in a frying pan, cook the venison for 5 mins, then turn over and cook for 3-5 mins more, depending on how rare you like it and the thickness of the meat (cook for 5-6 mins on each side for well done). Lift the meat from the pan and set aside to rest.

- Add the balsamic vinegar to the pan, then pour in the stock, redcurrant jelly and garlic. Stir over quite a high heat to blend everything together, then add the blackberries and carry on cooking until they soften. Serve with the venison, celeriac mash and broccoli.

Spiced Chicken With Rice & Crisp Red Onions

Ingredients

- 2 boneless skinless chicken breasts, about 140g/5oz each
- 1 tbsp sunflower oil
- 2 tsp curry powder
- 1 large red onion, thinly sliced
- 100g basmati rice
- 1 cinnamon stick
- pinch saffron
- 1 tbsp raisins
- 85g frozen pea
- 1 tbsp chopped mint and coriander
- 4 rounded tbsp low-fat natural yogurt

Method

- Heat oven to 190C/fan 170C/gas 5. Brush the chicken with 1 tsp oil, then sprinkle with curry powder. Toss the onion in the remaining oil. Put the chicken and onions in one layer in a roasting tin. Bake for 25 mins until the meat is cooked and the onions are crisp, stirring the onions halfway through the cooking time.

• Rinse the rice, then put in a pan with the cinnamon, saffron, salt to taste and 300ml water. Bring to the boil, stir once, add the raisins, cover. Gently cook for 10-12 mins until the rice is tender, adding the peas halfway through. Spoon the rice onto two plates, top with the chicken and scatter over the onions. Stir the herbs into the yogurt and season, if you like, before serving on the side.

Prawn Sweet Chilli Noodle Salad
Ingredients

- 3 nests medium egg noodles

- ½ large cucumber

- bunch spring onions, finely sliced

- 100g cherry tomato, halved

- 1 green chilli, deseeded, finely chopped

- 200g cooked king prawns, defrosted if frozen

- zest and juice 2 limes

- 4 tbsp sweet chilli sauce

- 100g baby spinach leaves

- 25g roasted cashew

Method

- Boil the noodles for 4 mins, then drain. Cool under running water, then drain again. Put into a large bowl, then using scissors, cut into shorter lengths.

- Halve cucumber lengthways, then scoop out the seeds. Slice into halfmoons and add to the noodles with the onions, tomatoes, chilli and prawns.

- Mix the lime zest, juice and chilli sauce to make a dressing and fold through noodles. Put a handful of spinach onto each serving plate, top with the noodles and cashews.

Chargrilled Turkey With Quinoa Tabbouleh & Tahini Dressing

Ingredients

- 200g quinoa

- ½ cucumber, cut into 1cm chunks

- 175g cherry tomato, halved

- 3 spring onions, finely sliced

- handful parsley, roughly chopped

- handful coriander, roughly chopped

- 1 tbsp olive oil, plus 1 tsp

- juice 1 lemon

- 4 turkey steaks

For the tahini dressing

- 1½ tbsp tahini paste

- 1½ tbsp low-fat yogurt

- juice ½ lemon

- ½ garlic clove, crushed

- ½ tsp clear honey

Method

- Tip the quinoa into a saucepan and pour over 600ml water. Cover with a lid and bring to the boil. Turn down and simmer until the water has evaporated (just as you'd cook rice) – about 20 mins. Take off the lid and leave to cool while you prepare the turkey and salad.

- Tip the cucumber, tomatoes, spring onions and herbs into a large mixing bowl. Pour over 1 tbsp olive oil and lemon juice, season well and mix everything together.

- Heat a griddle pan and, when smoking hot, rub the turkey steaks with 1 tsp olive oil. Cook for about 5 mins on each side, depending on thickness. Stir together all the dressing ingredients along with 3 tbsp water. Toss the quinoa together with the salad and arrange on plates. Cut the turkey into thick slices, pile up on the quinoa and drizzle over the dressing.

Chicken Korma

Ingredients

- 2 tbsp vegetable oil

- 2 medium onions, chopped

- 3 garlic cloves

- about 2cm piece fresh root ginger (to give you 2 tbsp finely chopped)

- 5 cardamom pods

- 1 cinnamon stick

- 600g boneless, skinless chicken breasts, cut into bite-size pieces
- 2 tsp ground coriander
- 1 ½ tsp garam masala
- ¼ tsp ground mace
- ½ tsp ground black pepper
- 150ml natural yogurt, not fridge cold
- 100ml full-fat milk
- 2 small green chillies, deseeded and shredded
- handful coriander leaves and stems, coursely chopped
- 1 tbsp flaked almonds, toasted
- 250g basmati rice, cooked with a generous pinch saffron

Method

- Heat 1 tbsp of the oil in a deep sauté pan or wok. Tip in the onions, then fry over a medium-high heat for about 12-15 mins, stirring occasionally, until a rich golden colour and the pan is sticky on the bottom. While they cook, chop the garlic and ginger. Make a slit down the length of each cardamom pod just deep enough to reveal the tiny seeds. Remove the onions from the heat. Transfer a third of them to a small blender along with the garlic, ginger and 2 tbsp water. Whizz together to make a paste that is as smooth as you can get it. Set aside.

- Return the onions in the pan to the heat, add the remaining oil, cardamom pods and cinnamon stick, then stir-fry for a couple of mins. Stir in the chicken, ground coriander, 1¼ tsp of the garam masala, mace and black pepper, then stir-fry for another 2 mins. Reserve 3 tbsp of the yogurt, then slowly start to add the rest, 1 tbsp at a time, stirring between each spoonful. When all the yogurt has gone in, stir in the oniony paste and stir-fry for 2-3 mins. Stir in 150ml water, then the milk. Bring to a boil, then simmer, covered, for 20 mins, scattering in the chillies for the final 5 mins, by which time the chicken should be very tender. Remove the cardamom pods and cinnamon. The flavours mellow all the more if refrigerated overnight. When gently reheating, splash in a little water if needed to slacken the korma sauce.

- Finish by stirring in the chopped coriander. Taste and add a little salt if you wish. Swirl in the reserved yogurt. Spoon the korma into bowls, scatter a few almonds over each portion with a sprinkling of the remaining garam masala. Serve the saffron rice on the side.

Oven-Baked Fish & Chips
Ingredients

- 800g/ 1lb 12 oz floury potato, scrubbed and cut into chips

- 2 tbsp olive oil

- 50g fresh breadcrumb

- zest 1 lemon

- 2 tbsp chopped flat-leaf parsley

- 4 x 140g/5oz thick sustainable white fish fillets

- 200g/ 7oz cherry tomato

Method

- Heat oven to 220C/200C fan/gas 7. Pat chips dry on kitchen paper, then lay in a single layer on a large baking tray. Drizzle with half the olive oil and season with salt. Cook for 40 mins, turning after 20 mins, so they cook evenly.

- Mix the breadcrumbs with the lemon zest and parsley, then season well. Top the cod evenly with the breadcrumb mixture, then drizzle .0with the remaining oil. Put in a roasting tin with the cherry tomatoes, then bake in the oven for the final 10 mins of the chips' cooking time.

Chicken, Edamame & Ginger Pilaf
Ingredients

- 2 tbsp vegetable oil
- 1 onion, thinly sliced
- thumb-sized piece ginger, grated
- 1 red chilli, deseeded and finely sliced
- 3 skinless chicken breasts, cut into bite-sized pieces
- 250g basmati rice
- 600ml vegetable stock
- 100g frozen edamame / soya beans
- coriander leaves and fat-free Greek yoghurt (optional), to serve

Method

- Heat the oil in a medium saucepan, then add the onion, ginger and chilli, along with some seasoning. Cook for 5 mins, then add the chicken and rice. Cook for 2 mins more, then add the stock and bring to the boil. Turn the heat to low, cover and cook for 8-10 mins until the rice is just cooked. During the final 3 mins of cooking, add the edamame beans. Sprinkle some coriander leaves on top and serve with a dollop of Greek yogurt, if you like.

Spiced Turkey With Bulgur & Pomegranate Salad
Ingredients

- 2 tbsp each chopped dill, parsley and mint

- zest and juice 1 lemon

- 1 tbsp harissa paste

- 500g/1lb 2oz turkey breast fillets

- 2 tbsp white wine or water

- 250g pack bulgur wheat or a mix- we used quinoa and bulgur mix)

- 2 tomatoes, chopped

- ½ cucumber, diced

- 100g pack pomegranate seeds

Method

- Heat oven to 200C/180C fan/gas 6. Mix together half the herbs, half the lemon zest and juice, and all the harissa with some seasoning. Rub the turkey in the marinade and leave for 5 mins (or up to 24 hrs. in the fridge).

- Lay out a large sheet of foil. Put the turkey and marinade, and wine or water, on top, then cover with another layer of foil, fold and crimp the edges to seal. Transfer the parcel to a tray, then bake for 30 mins until cooked through.

- Meanwhile, make the salad. Cook the bulgur following pack instructions. Drain, then mix with the remaining herbs, lemon zest and juice, plus the tomatoes, cucumber and pomegranate seeds. Slice the turkey and serve on top of the salad with the foil parcel juices poured on top.

Chilli Pepper Pumpkin With Asian Veg

Ingredients

- 1 small pumpkin or ½ butternut squash, cut into chunks (seeds removed), no need to peel

- 2 tsp sunflower or vegetable oil

- 1 tsp each mild chilli powder and five spice powder

- 175g thin-stemmed broccoli

- 175g bok choi, quartered

- 2 tbsp low-sodium soy sauce

- 2 tbsp rice wine vinegar

- 1 tbsp honey

- 1 lime, ½ juice, ½ cut into wedges

- few coriander leaves

Method

- Heat oven to 220C/200C fan/gas 7. Toss the pumpkin in the oil, then sprinkle on the chilli powder, five-spice, 1 tsp black pepper and a pinch of salt, and mix well. Tip into a roasting tray in a single layer and cook for 25-30 mins until tender and starting to caramelise around the edges.

- About 5 mins before the pumpkin is cooked, heat a wok or large frying pan and add the broccoli plus 1-2 tbsp water. Cook for 2-3 mins, then add the bok choi, soy, vinegar and honey, and cook for a further 2-3 mins until the veg is tender. Add the lime juice, then divide between 2 plates with the pumpkin, coriander leaves and lime wedges.

Summer Pea Pasta
Ingredients

- 3 tbsp olive oil

- 3 fat garlic cloves, finely chopped

- 1 red chilli, deseeded and finely chopped

- zest 2 lemons

- 400g pasta

- 200g fresh or frozen peas

- 20g pack basil

Method

- Heat 1 tbsp oil in a frying pan and cook the garlic and chilli for a couple of mins until very lightly golden. Stir in the zest.

- Cook the pasta, adding the peas for the final 2 mins. Drain, then tip everything back into the saucepan. Tip in the garlic, chilli and lemon, scraping in any bits stuck to the pan. Tear in the basil, season and add the remaining olive oil. Stir well.

Miso Steak
Ingredients

- 2 tbsp brown miso paste

- 1 tbsp dry sherry or sake

- 1 tbsp caster sugar

- 2 crushed garlic cloves

- 300g/11oz lean steak

- baby spinach, sliced cucumber, celery, radish and toasted sesame seeds, to serve

Method

- Tip the miso paste, Sherry or sake, sugar and garlic into a sealable food bag. Season with a generous grinding of black pepper, then squash it all together until completely mixed. Add the steak, gently massage the marinade into the steak until completely coated, then seal the bag. Pop the bag into the fridge and leave for at least 1 hr, but up to 2 days is fine.

- To cook, heat a heavy-based frying pan, griddle pan or barbecue until very hot. Wipe the excess marinade off the steak, then sear for 3 mins on each side for medium-rare or a few mins longer if you prefer the meat more cooked. Set aside for 1 min to rest. Carve the beef into thick slices and serve with a crunchy salad made with the spinach, cucumber, celery, radish and sesame seeds.

Low-Fat Roasties
Ingredients

- 800g roasting potatoes, quartered
- 1 garlic clove, sliced
- 200ml vegetable stock (from a cube is fine)
- 2 tbsp olive oil

Method

- Heat oven to 200C/fan 180C/gas 6. Put the potatoes and garlic in a roasting tin. Pour over the stock, then brush the tops of the potatoes with half the olive oil. Season, then cook for 50 mins. Brush with the remaining oil and cook

10-15 mins more until the stock is absorbed and the potatoes have browned and cooked through.

Ceviche

Ingredients

- 500g firm white fish fillets, such as haddock, halibut or pollack, skinned and thinly sliced
- juice 8 limes (250ml/9fl oz), plus extra wedges to serve
- 1 red onion, sliced into rings
- handful pitted green olives, finely chopped
- 2-3 green chillies, finely chopped
- 2-3 tomatoes, seeded and chopped into 2cm pieces
- bunch coriander, roughly chopped
- 2 tbsp extra-virgin olive oil
- good pinch caster sugar
- tortilla chips, to serve

Method

- In a large glass bowl, combine the fish, lime juice and onion. The juice should completely cover the fish; if not, add a little more. Cover with cling film and place in the fridge for 1 hr 30 mins.

- Remove the fish and onion from the lime juice (discard the juice) and place in a bowl. Add the olives, chilies, tomatoes, coriander and olive oil, stir gently, then season with a good pinch of salt and sugar. This can be made a couple of hours in advance and stored in the fridge. Serve with tortilla chips to scoop up the ceviche and enjoy with a glass of cold beer.

Mushroom & Thyme Risotto

Ingredients

- 1 tbsp olive oil

- 350g chestnut mushrooms, sliced

- 100g quinoa

- 1l hot vegetable stock

- 175g risotto rice

- handful of thyme leaves

- handful of grated parmesan or vegetarian alternative

- 50g bag rocket, to serve

Method

- Heat the oil in a medium pan, sauté the mushrooms for 2-3 mins, then stir in the quinoa. Keeping the vegetable stock warm in a separate pan on a low heat, add a ladle of the stock and stir until absorbed. Stir in the rice and repeat again with the stock, until all the stock has been used up and the rice and quinoa are tender and cooked.

- Stir in the thyme leaves, then divide between four plates or bowls. Serve topped with grated parmesan and rocket leaves.

Mango & Passion Fruit Meringue Roulade
Ingredients

- 3 large egg whites

- 175g caster sugar

- 1 level tsp corn flour

- 1 tsp malt vinegar

- 1 tsp vanilla extract

- icing sugar, to dust
- 200g fat-free Greek yogurt
- 1 large ripe mango, peeled, stoned and diced
- 4 passion fruits, pulp only
- icing sugar (optional) and a few physalis, to decorate
- raspberry sauce, to serve

Method

- Preheat the oven to 150C/ gas 2/fan 130C. Line a 33x23cm swiss roll tin with non-stick baking parchment. Beat the egg whites with an electric whisk until frothy and doubled in bulk. Slowly whisk in the caster sugar until thick and shiny. Mix the corn flour, vinegar and vanilla extract, then whisk into the egg whites.

- Spoon into the tin and level the surface carefully, so you don't push out the air. Bake for 30 minutes until the meringue surface is just firm.

- Remove from the oven and cover with damp greaseproof paper for 10 minutes. Dust another sheet of greaseproof paper with icing sugar. Discard the damp paper and turn the meringue out on to the sugarcoated paper. Peel off the lining paper, then spread yogurt over the meringue and scatter with mango and passion fruit. Use the paper to roll up the roulade from one short end. Keep the join underneath. Sift a little icing sugar on top if you like, decorate with physalis and serve with raspberry sauce.

Chicken With Lemon & Courgette Couscous
Ingredients

- 200g couscous

- 400ml chicken stock

- 2 tbsp olive oil

- 4 courgettes, grated

- 2 lemons, 1 halved, 1 cut into wedges

- 2 boneless, skinless chicken breasts

Method

- Tip the couscous into a large bowl and pour over the stock. Cover and leave for 10 mins until fluffy and all the stock has been absorbed. Heat 1 tbsp oil and fry the courgettes until softened and crisping at the edges. Tip into the couscous, then stir in with plenty of seasoning and a good squeeze of lemon juice from one of the halves.

- Halve the chicken breasts horizontally and put each piece on a sheet of cling film. Cover with another sheet and beat each piece out with a rolling pin to make it thinner. Season. Heat the remaining oil in a large pan and fry the chicken for about 2 mins on each side until cooked through. Squeeze over the juice from the other lemon half and serve with the couscous and lemon wedges on the side.

Thai Red Duck With Sticky Pineapple Rice
Ingredients

- 2 duck breasts, skin removed and discarded

- 1 tbsp Thai red curry paste

- zest and juice 1 lime, plus extra wedges to serve

- 140g jasmine rice

- 125ml light coconut milk, from a can

- 140g frozen peas

- 50g beansprouts

- ½ red onion, diced

- 100g fresh pineapple, cubed

- 1 red chilli, deseeded and finely chopped

- ¼ small pack coriander, stalks finely chopped, leaves roughly chopped

Method

- Sit a duck breast between 2 sheets of cling film on a chopping board. Use a rolling pin to bash the duck until it is 0.5cm thick. Repeat with the other breast, then put them both in a dish. Mix the curry paste with the lime zest and juice, and rub all over the duck. Leave to marinate at room temperature for 20 mins.

- Meanwhile, tip the rice into a small saucepan with some salt. Pour over the coconut milk with 150ml water. Bring to a simmer, then cover the pan, turn the heat down low and cook for 5 more mins. Stir in the peas, then cover, turn the heat off and leave for another 10 mins. Check the rice - all the liquid should be absorbed and the rice cooked through. Boil the kettle, put the beansprouts and red onion in a colander and pour over a kettleful of boiling water. Stir the beansprouts and onion into the rice with the pineapple, chilli and coriander stalks, and some more salt if it needs it, and put the lid back on to keep warm.

- Heat a griddle pan and cook the duck for 1-2 mins each side or until cooked to your liking. Slice the duck, stir most of the coriander leaves through the rice with a fork to fluff up, and serve alongside the duck, scattered with the remaining coriander.

Prawn, Fennel & Rocket Risotto
Ingredients

- 1.2l vegetable stock

- 1 tbsp olive oil

- 1 onion, finely chopped

- 1 large garlic clove, finely chopped

- 1 small fennel bulb, cored and finely chopped

- 300g risotto rice

- 300g peeled raw king prawns

- 1 lemon, ½ zested and 1 tbsp juice

- 70g bag rocket

Method

- Put the stock in a large saucepan, bring to the boil, then lower to a simmer. Meanwhile, heat the oil in a large saucepan. Add the onion, garlic and fennel, and cook on a low heat for 10 mins until the vegetables have softened but not colored. Add the rice and stir for 2 mins until the grains are hot and making crackling sounds. Increase the heat to medium and start adding the stock, a ladleful at a time, stirring constantly and making sure the stock has absorbed into the rice before adding the next ladleful.

- When the rice is almost cooked, add the prawns, lemon zest and some seasoning. Continue adding stock and cooking for another 3-4 mins until the prawns are pink and the rice is cooked. Remove from the heat and stir through the rocket and lemon juice. Check the seasoning, leave the risotto to sit in the pan for 2 mins, then serve.

Red Lentil, Chickpea & Chilli Soup
Ingredients

- 2 tsp cumin seeds

- large pinch chilli flakes

- 1 tbsp olive oil

- 1 red onion, chopped

- 140g red split lentils

- 850ml vegetable stock or water

- 400g can tomatoes, whole or chopped

- 200g can chickpeas or ½ a can, drained and rinsed (freeze leftovers)

- small bunch coriander, roughly chopped (save a few leaves, to serve)

- 4 tbsp 0% Greek yogurt, to serve

Method

- Heat a large saucepan and dry-fry 2 tsp cumin seeds and a large pinch of chilli flakes for 1 min, or until they start to jump around the pan and release their aromas.

- Add 1 tbsp olive oil and 1 chopped red onion, and cook for 5 mins.

- Stir in 140g red split lentils, 850ml vegetable stock or water and a 400g can tomatoes, then bring to the boil. Simmer for 15 mins until the lentils have softened.

- Whizz the soup with a stick blender or in a food processor until it is a rough purée, pour back into the pan and add a 200g can drained and rinsed chickpeas.

- Heat gently, season well and stir in a small bunch of chopped coriander, reserving a few leaves to serve. Finish with 4 tbsp 0% Greek yogurt and extra coriander leaves.

Granola

Serves 8, Prep time: 10 minutes, Cook time: 6 hours on low, 3 hours on high.

When you think low-carb, granola usually isn't at the top of the list. And most people think store-bought granola is healthy, so they don't make their own. Unfortunately, a lot of store-bought granola is covered in—guess what? sugar. Lucky for you, this low-carb version is really easy to make (and it tastes great), and you get to be in control of the ingredients, ensuring they are natural with no added fillers.

Ingredients

- 2½ cups almonds

- ¼ cup unsweetened coconut flakes

- ½ cup dried berries

- ¼ cup chia seeds

- 1 teaspoon cinnamon

- ½ teaspoon salt

- ¼ teaspoon nutmeg

- ¼ cup coconut oil

- 1 teaspoon vanilla

Direction

- Coat the sides of a slow cooker generously with cooking spray.

- Add the almonds, coconut flakes, dried berries, chia seeds, cinnamon, salt, and nutmeg to the slow cooker.

- In a medium bowl, melt the coconut oil. Whisk in the vanilla.

- Pour the mixture into the slow cooker, stirring to make sure all the ingredients are moistened.

- Lay a small towel or 2 paper towels in between the slow cooker and the lid to create a barrier. This will prevent the condensation from dripping on the granola while it cooks. It's important to catch the condensation or you will end up with soggy granola.

- Cook mixture on low for 6 hours or on high for 3 hours.

- Transfer the granola to a baking sheet to cool.

Cauliflower Mac and Cheese

Serves 6, Prep time: 10 minutes, Cook time: 4 to 6 hours on low, 2 to 3 hours on high

Macaroni and cheese lovers rejoice! When you swap out the pasta and use cauliflower, you're left with a low-carb taste sensation that is creamy and filling. It makes great leftovers and the kids will like it, too. If the sauce seems too thick after it's finished cooking, stir in a little water or vegetable broth.

Ingredients

- 2 medium heads cauliflower, cut into small florets

- 1 small onion, diced

- 3 cups Cheese Sauce

Direction

- Coat a slow cooker generously with cooking spray.

- Add the cauliflower and onion to the slow cooker.

- Pour the cheese sauce over the top.

- Cook on low for 4 to 6 hours or on high for 2 to 3 hours, or until the cauliflower is tender.

Balsamic And Bacon Vegetable Medley

Serves 4, Prep time: 15 minutes, Cook time: 4 to 6 hours on low, 2 to 3 hours on high.

Here is a side dish perfect for summer, when these vegetables will be at their freshest and most flavorful. By cooking in a slow cooker, you don't need to stand over a hot stove. Feel free to swap in whatever veggies you like the best. And it's never wrong to add a little extra bacon.

Ingredients

- 8 ounces bacon, cooked and crumbled

- 1 small onion, chopped
- 2 bell peppers, seeded and chopped
- 3 ounces carrots, peeled and chopped
- 3 ounces green beans, cut into 1-inch pieces
- 3 ounces Brussels sprouts, trimmed and halved
- 3 ounces beets, peeled and chopped
- 3 ounces summer squash or zucchini, chopped
- ¼ cup water
- 1 tablespoon extra-virgin olive oil
- 2 tablespoons balsamic vinegar

Direction

- Coat a slow cooker generously with cooking spray.

- Add the bacon, onion, bell peppers, carrots, green beans, Brussels sprouts, beets, and squash to the slow cooker.

- In a small bowl, mix together the water, olive oil, and vinegar to make a sauce. Pour it over the top of the vegetables.

- Cook on low for 4 to 6 hours or on high for 2 to 3 hours, or until Brussels sprouts are tender.

Garden Vegetable Soup

Serves 4, Prep time: 10 minutes, Cook time: 6 to 8 hours on low, 3 to 4 hours on high.

Grab your favorite vegetables for this super easy soup that is friendly for almost any healthy eating lifestyle: paleo, Whole30, vegetarian, vegan—it's a real diet pleaser. I love the combination of vegetables I've included below, but don't let that fence you in. Swap in whatever you find in the store that's fresh and low-carb. Try yellow squash instead of zucchini, or asparagus instead of green beans. Choose sturdy vegetables that won't turn to mush during the long cook time.

Ingredients

- 4 cups Vegetable Broth or store-bought low-sodium vegetable broth
- 1 (15-ounce) can low-sodium or no-salt-added diced tomatoes
- 2 small zucchini, diced

- 2 carrots, peeled and chopped
- 4 ounces green beans, chopped
- 4 ounces kale, chopped
- 1 onion, diced
- 1 bell pepper, seeded and diced
- 2 garlic cloves, minced
- 1 tablespoon Italian seasoning
- ½ teaspoon salt
- ¼ teaspoon freshly ground black pepper
- 1 bay leaf

Direction

- Add the broth, tomatoes, zucchini, carrots, green beans, kale, onion, bell pepper, garlic, Italian seasoning, salt, black pepper, and bay leaf to a slow cooker.
- Cook on low for 6 to 8 hours or on high for 3 to 4 hours, or until vegetables are soft.
- Remove the bay leaf prior to serving.

French Onion Soup

Serves 4, Prep time: 10 minutes, Cook time: 6 to 8 hours on low, 3 to 4 hours on high

French onion soup is an all-time favorite of mine. I've never really been a big bread person, so this low-carb version is right up my alley. If you sauté the onions in a little butter on medium-low for about 10 minutes, your soup will have a richer, deeper flavor, so if you have the time, do that. But if you don't, never fear—it will still taste terrific. Slice the onions as thin as you can; if you have a mandoline, this is a good time to use it.

Ingredient

- 4 cups low-sodium beef broth

- 4 medium white onions, sliced as thin as possible

- 2 tablespoons unsalted butter

- 2 garlic cloves, minced

- ½ teaspoon salt

- ¼ teaspoon freshly ground black pepper

- 1 bay leaf

- 4 (1-ounce) slices provolone cheese

Direction

- Add the broth, onions, butter, garlic, salt, pepper, and bay leaf to a slow cooker. Stir to mix well.

- Cook on low for 6 to 8 hours or on high for 3 to 4 hours.

- Preheat the oven to broil.

- Ladle the soup into 4 oven-safe soup bowls and place on a baking sheet. Place 1 slice of provolone over the soup in each bowl, and broil for 1 minute, or until the cheese melts.

Blueberry Muffin Cake

Serves 10, Prep time: 15 minutes, Cook time: 4 to 6 hours on low, 2 to 3 hours on high.

Is this a cake or a muffin? It's both. Serve this sweet, keto-friendly blueberry treat as an after-dinner dessert or as part of your next brunch spread.

Ingredient

- 3 cups almond flour

- ½ cup 2% fat plain Greek yogurt

- ¼ cup powdered erythritol sweetener of your choice
- 3 large eggs
- 2 to 3 teaspoons grated lemon zest
- 1½ teaspoons baking powder
- 1 teaspoon vanilla extract
- ½ teaspoon baking soda
- ¼ teaspoon salt
- 1 cup fresh or frozen blueberries

Direction

- Coat a slow cooker generously with cooking spray.
- In a large bowl, mix together the almond flour, yogurt, erythritol, eggs, lemon zest, baking powder, vanilla, baking soda, and salt until well blended. Carefully fold in the blueberries.
- Pour the batter into the slow cooker.
- Place a paper towel between the slow cooker and the lid to cut down on any condensation that develops. Cook on

low for 4 to 6 hours or on high for 2 to 3 hours, or until a toothpick inserted in the center comes out clean.

Pecan Cookie

Serves 8, Prep time: 10 minutes, Cook time: 4 to 6 hours on low, 2 to 3 hours on high

This will remind you of a buttery pecan sandie, but you can enjoy it guilt-free. It's another great option if you're following a keto diet, too.

Ingredient

- 1¼ cup almond flour
- ⅔ cup powdered erythritol sweetener of your choice
- ⅓ cup chopped pecans
- 1 large egg
- 5 tablespoons unsalted butter, at room temperature
- 1 tablespoon coconut flour
- 1 teaspoon baking powder
- ½ teaspoon vanilla extract

Direction

- Coat a slow cooker generously with cooking spray.

- In a large bowl, mix together the almond flour, erythritol, pecans, egg, butter, coconut flour, baking powder, and vanilla until well blended. Pour the batter into the slow cooker.

- Place a paper towel between the slow cooker and the lid to cut down on any condensation that develops. Cook on low for 4 to 6 hours or on high for 2 to 3 hours, or until a toothpick inserted in the center comes out clean.

Made in the USA
Columbia, SC
29 September 2023